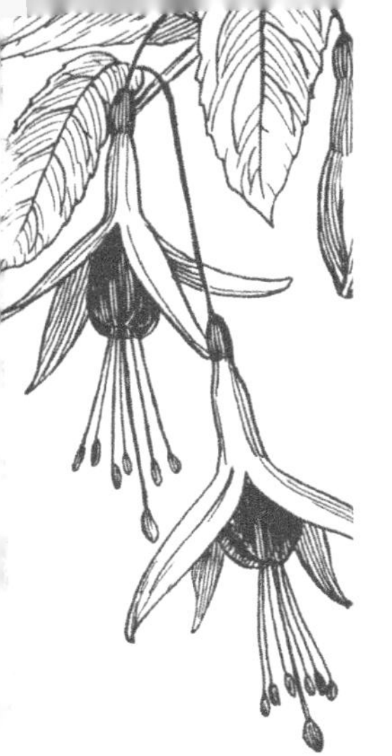

Watering the Soul

A 91-Day Purposeful Self-Care Journal for Caregivers

Keli Gooch, LPC/MHSP

Watering the Soul, by Keli Gooch

Written by: Keli Gooch
First Printing, 2019
ISBN: 9781094923925

Visit the author's website, at keligooch.com.

Disclaimer: The information and prompts in this journal should not be used as a replacement for individual therapy or treatment by a mental health professional. While self-help information is useful, it is not a substitute for personal professional advice.
If you are currently receiving treatment, please consult with your therapist or doctor before utilizing this journal.

Dedicated to my sister Krystal & my CCMM sisters:

for incessantly helping me water my own soul

PREFACE.

When we moved into our home 7 years ago, our grass was in critical condition. Literally- our lawn was more brown than green and full of alien-like weeds. Whenever I strolled across the grass, it made a crunchy sound, crisp like rippled potato chips. I remember going out many times to play ball or enjoy the sun with my daughter. It was always fun, but the ground was so noisy and was definitely unpleasant to walk on barefooted.

So, we decided to invest in professional lawn care services. We signed an agreement in which every month, professionals would come out and spray our yard to get rid of all the crazy weeds. It took many treatments, but after several months, the weeds began to dissipate. Our grass slowly transformed in a lush, bright forest green. The crunchy exterior of our grass no longer existed, and what we were left with were soft blades that would blow and move on a windy day.

Now, each time the Lawn Care Professionals treated our yard, they left very specific instructions about watering the grass. Our specialist told us if we didn't water our lawn regularly, we could eventually start to develop dry spots or dry patches in our grass. He said, "this is especially true in the summer time. The summer heat can cause real damage to the grass."

Truthfully, my husband and I didn't really want to make the investment in the lawn care services, but without it, our grass would have remained in its barren, desert-like shape.

My friend, YOU may feel just like our grass did 7 years ago. Dry, brittle, hard-on-the-outside, and just plain bare. The heat and stress of your life may have caused dry spots.

Maybe you help take care of a parent with dementia, or a complex child, or maybe you are a professional caretaker or home health nurse with the invaluable job of taking care of someone else's loved one.

Research has shown that caregivers, while viewing their job as enjoyable and rewarding, also are at risk for health problems, as well as mental health difficulties.

As caregivers, we sometimes forget about ourselves. We live in "ON" mode and work tirelessly non-stop. We stay armed with medical knowledge and we are our loved-ones' fiercest advocates. This journal is an investment in YOU. Please read this next sentence carefully.

You MUST take time to care for yourself (and that does NOT include the 10 minute alone trip you took to your favorite chain store). I mean, meaningful, purposeful time focused on you. This includes an examination into who you are, who you want to be, and discovering your own secret hopes and dreams.

This journal is broken down into a series of prompts, followed by actionable steps. Ideally you might start on Sunday, so these actionable steps could be done over the weekend, but feel free to start on any day you want.
Also... are you paying attention?

DO NOT- skim over the actions. They are important to you and your own mental health.
By investing in this book, I assume you probably recognize the importance of taking care of yourself.
I hope that as you go through each page, you recognize what a true gift you are, and that the blades of your heart and soul soften, and start to turn forest green too.

Keli Gooch

Week 1

Births & Beginnings

Birth of My Role as Caregiver

We have already established that you are a caregiver (pretty sure that's the reason you got the journal!). Here is my story and how I unexpectedly became a caregiver.

Have you ever been in such a state of shock where you felt as though your heart stopped beating, and you felt like you had stopped breathing? The air in the room felt stifled and in the deepest part of your ear, all you could hear is a high-pitched, screeching sound?

I have to be honest. That is how I felt on the day my daughter was born. You have to understand that my 22-year-old brain was vastly different from my now 39-year-old brain.

At the age of 22, and in my final year of college, I became pregnant. In the beginning, my pregnancy was normal. All of my baby's measurements were normal, except for a bit of extra amniotic fluid. I figured she just had more water to swim around in. I passed my Alpha Fetoprotein blood test as well. (This test examines a protein in the blood that is produced by a fetus- these levels can be used to look for congenital issues such as Down Syndrome).

Later on in my pregnancy, and 3 months before I was to graduate with my BS in psychology, I began to develop preeclampsia, so I was put on bed rest. The week of my Comprehensive Exams, I was scheduled for a routine appointment. My cousin drove me and we made a pit stop at Chick-Fil-A.

After finishing eating my sandwich loaded with pickles, I walked in for my routine exam. My awesome nurse proceeded to attach the heart monitor to my now huge belly. She then printed out of copy of my baby's heartbeat, and then another nurse came in. My doctor then came in to examine me. With a look of concern, he told me "Your baby's heart rate is decelerating. We need you to go to the hospital immediately for an emergency C-section."

I remember being afraid, so I called my mom to meet me. As I lay down, I remember having fear about the C-section, but also excitement about meeting my baby girl. After my C-section, I remember looking at my mom's face after seeing my baby. She looked really worried. Once I returned To my room from recovery, I was told that my baby had to be rushed to a larger hospital in a neighboring city because her heart had stopped beating 3 times due to a possible heart defect.

Tears begin to flow, but I knew I needed to be strong for her. Later that evening, I received a call from that hospital with the news, "Your daughter has Down Syndrome. Down Syndrome means that she won't be very smart. It may take her longer to walk and to talk. When she grows up she may be able to work at McDonald's and push a mop."

And that's how my caregiver role began. I was given so much negative information when my daughter was born. I never imagined how much she would enrich my life, and that with work, how my life could turn out to be amazing.

This week, let's focus on how your caregiver role began.

I sure hope it wasn't as rocky as mine!

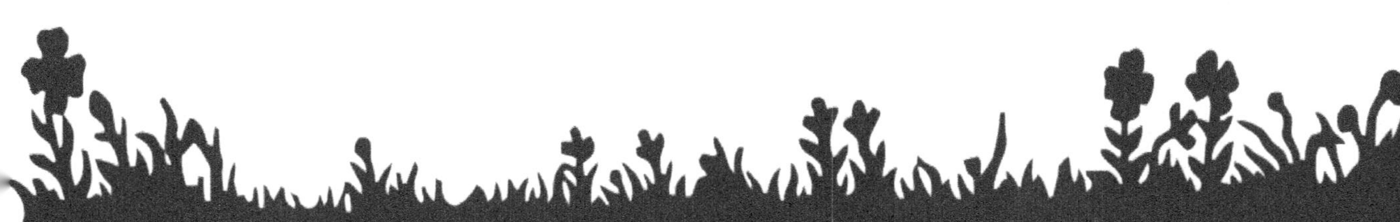

Day 1

Imagine you are meeting someone new for the first time. Tell your story of exactly how you came to be a caregiver. How did you feel in the beginning?

Day 2

How are you feeling about your role as caregiver today? Express yourself honestly and write down every feeling you are experiencing at this moment.

Day 3

What is your biggest obstacle right now? Write down any road blocks you are having today and be sure to jot down how these obstacles affect you.

Day 4

What's your biggest frustration today? Does it include your situation or are internal factors the source?

Day 5

Today, focus on the negative thoughts you might have. What type of negative, false thoughts run through your head? Are there any truth to those thoughts?

Day 6

Jot down every positive aspect about your role as caregiver.

Day 7- Sprinkle today with.......

Calm

It's your first purposeful self-care day. Today you will schedule a time next week to sit and talk and drink your favorite coffee (or tea if coffee isn't your thing) with a friend or by yourself. Oh and No excuses! Can't find a sitter or someone to watch your loved one? Have coffee time in your house!

Week 2

Change

"Nothing in life is as constant and consistent as change."

Day 8

If there was one thing you could change about your life, what would you change?

Day 9

What is the hardest choice you have ever had to make? Name several hard choices or decisions.

Day 10

Look back at all the choices you wrote down yesterday. Make a list of things you wish you could have done differently.

Day 11

Today look back at the choices and decisions you have had to make. Make a list of things that were in your control vs. things you feel were out of your control.

Day 12

Often when we are caregivers, our circle of friends can change. Jot down how your friends have changed since you became a caregiver.

Day 13

How have your finances changed since you have been a caregiver? Are there things you need to change? Do you need to make a budget and stick with it?

Day 14- Sprinkle today with.......

Change

Look back at your list of things you wish you could change from earlier this week. Is there anything that IS in your control and that you do have the power to change? Pick 1 person to be accountable to and share 1 thing you will work on changing.

Week 3

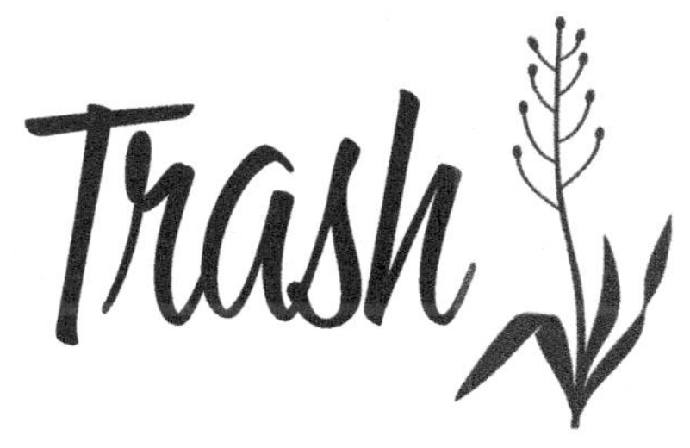

Throw it Away

I think in life, sometimes we just accept what is, because it is easier for us to deal with and comprehend- a form of coping. At times, though, hoping is utterly exhausting. It isn't that you give up, it's just that acceptance is often easier to live with and easier for the brain to understand and compartmentalize.

My 16-year old daughter Tayler has Down Syndrome, as well as hypothyroidism, sleep difficulties, and hyperinsulemia, but she is still pretty healthy.

However, she is unable to communicate and is considered non-verbal. Sign Language has not been an option for us because it requires fine motor skills that she has difficulty with.

She makes noises that sometimes get stares, and she has occasionally said "go" and "hey," but has never uttered a full sentence.

Her amazing teachers told me Tayler has been trying to form words, but I wasn't quite prepared for what happened one night after Sunday dinner.

I had just made a meal of baked chicken coated with an unmentioned dressing. Nothing quite special. The cooked chicken rested quietly in a metal pan, with a simple salad alongside it.

After dinner, my husband let the leftover chicken cool before returning it to its home in the refrigerator. As I was leaving the room, I heard my husband say, "Tayler, what are you doing with that tray?"

Tayler lightly walked with both hands cupped on either side of the tray. I glanced quickly as she ended her stroll at our garbage can. She tilted the worn metal tray slightly and said,

"THROW IT AWAY."

She then handed the tray to my husband and casually walked away. My husband let out a huge, uproarious laugh.

I simply stared in disbelief and shock.

I never imaged that chicken (that honestly wasn't very great) would produce spontaneous speech.

The thoughts in my head included shock, sprinkled with confusion, topped with a slight offense (The chicken wasn't THAT bad). I also felt complete and utter pride and joy.

SO I THREW IT AWAY.

She did have a point.

This journey as a mom is full of unexpected surprises and turns. But Tayler was correct- I needed to throw some things away.

And maybe you should take my daughter's advice too.

Day 15

What are some strict timelines you have set in your head? Do you need to be more lenient and change them? Are you rigid and set in these timelines?

Day 16

Do you have self-doubt? Today write about areas in your life where you need to remove self-doubt.

Day 17

Today think about fears you need to trash. Are any of those fears irrational? Do you struggle with anxiety about those fears?

Day 18

This is a hard one. Write about the hurt you have felt in the past. Are you able to forgive at this point in your life? Share some past hurts you may need to trash.

Day 19

Write about the anger you feel or have felt in the past. Where does (did) the anger stem from? Share what angers you and how you can throw it away.

Day 20

Today- write down all the unsolicited advice you have received. Even from well-meaning individuals, are there any opinions you need to trash?

Day 21- Sprinkle today with.......

Trash

Okay, so let someone else take your garbage bags out today! I need you to treat yourself to dinner. Make it yourself or go out to eat- as long as YOU enjoy it and as long as it's not gross chicken!

Week 4

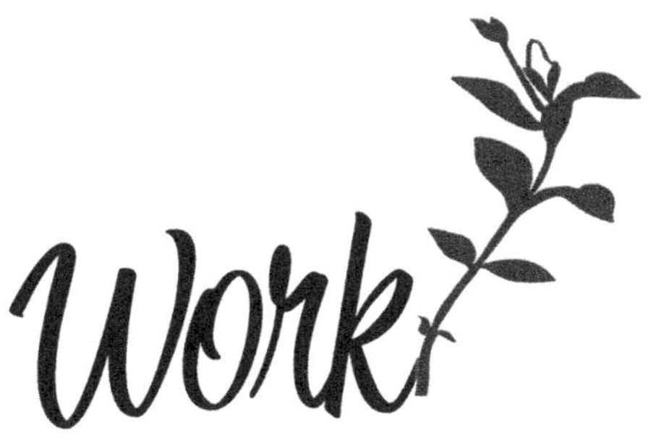

"Never start your day-
wishing it were time for bed."
- said no Caregiver ever

Day 22

Do you work outside of your home? If so, what are your personal career goals?

Day 23

Today, focus on general goals. Write down 5 long-term goals.

Day 24

Looking back at your long-term goals, now break each goal down into short-term goals- i.e. two short-term goals for every long-term goal.

Day 25

If you work outside of the home, what would you most like to change about your career?

Day 26

Do you have any regrets about your career life?

Day 27

Today- write down 5 things you would do career-wise if you were risky and felt brave?

Day 28- Sprinkle today with.......

A New Network

Today's challenge is to connect with someone on your job or in your career field. You have already written down your goals for the week- Be bold! You'd be surprised how great it feels to meet new people. And- if you don't work outside the home, venture out and connect with someone who shares the same hobbies.

Week 5

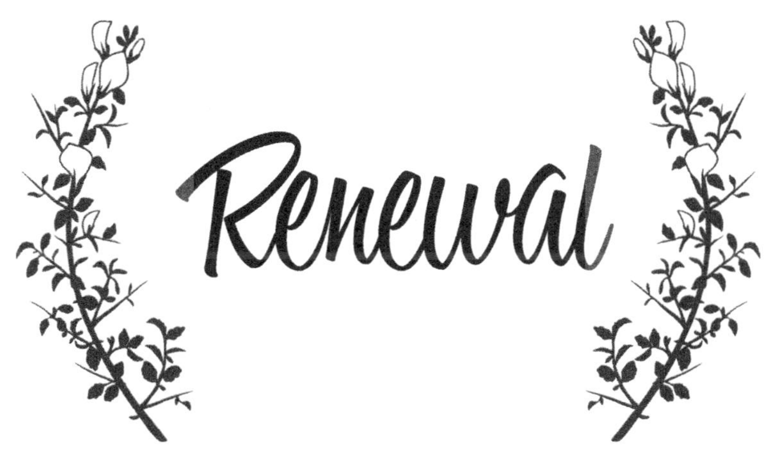

Out in the beautiful Serengeti, I hear the light gallop of cleft hooves. As the sound approaches, it becomes louder. That gallop soon turns into a full blown sprint and before I realize it, whatever created that sound has vanished.
A stately rhino? No.
A startled zebra?Hardly.
It's the sound of my preschooler running through my house. I sit and wonder in awe at this beautiful little creation who has completely transformed my life.
I want to chase her, but the cramp that just reached my calf muscle stops me.
And I am suddenly reminded....
I am a Mid-Life mom.

If the sudden urge to get a random tattoo didn't clue me in, the fact I now prefer to be in bed by 9 pm (on weekdays AND weekends), and the strong desire to binge-watch movies on Netflix rather than actually go to a movie theater should have made it completely clear. I've watched the young mothers gather at the after-school pick-up line dressed in their cute outfits or athletic wear and thought- I'm the "old" mom. They never cheat on their low-fat, no carb diets, hit the gym 5 times each week and still have time to get fully made up- hair and all.
Meanwhile, I cancelled my gym membership 2 weeks ago, stress-ate a delicious donut just now, and did my best to quickly tie my hair up into a top-knot using a stretched-out ponytail holder I found on the floor of my car to keep it out of my face while loading groceries and making my way to the next errand I have to run.

The beautiful truth is, however, I wouldn't trade this motherhood thing for anything in the world. I LOVE being over 30 because I understand SO many things now. As I enter into the cusp of a new chapter, standing on the brink of 40, motherhood is quite different for me this time. I was 22 when I had Tayler, and I was 34 with my second child. There are several noticeable differences.

Here are my secret confessions of my reality as a Mid-Life mom:

1. Sometimes I sit and stare at large piles in my home.
I stare at the piles of laundry, piles of mail, or the piles of half-dressed Barbies. As a Mid-Life mom, I am comfortable with just gazing at my multiple piles. I usually end up staring because...

2. I no longer care about having a "perfect" home.
I am comfortable with my weary couch, and those who enter should expect to see that my home is "lived-in." You receive no promises of perfect order when you arrive at my house unannounced. If you expect perfection, I suggest calling first and my husband and I will scramble to clean. Maybe.

3. Sometimes I don't cook. A lot of times- I don't cook.
When I first had second child, we ate organic everything. Organic kale, grass-fed beef, even juiced fresh vegetables like collards. But life hit.
With a picky preschooler, working 2 jobs to pay off debt, and a mother who is beautifully aging, my priorities have shifted and meals need to be convenient.
The energy to scoop spaghetti squash out of its shell is gone.
The zeal and extra energy to cook 6 days a week no longer exists and since I'm a midlife mom, I could care less if you judge me.

4. Opinions don't matter much anymore.
Whether its parenting advice, suggestions for my attire, or the latest shoe trends... I live and wear what works for me. It's not that I don't value my friends' opinions, but I have an innate determination to live this life with minimal regrets. I refuse to waste precious time mewling over the opinions of others, and I take unsolicited advice with a grain of salt. A very small grain of salt.

5. I'm determined to do things that scare me.
I am determined to push my limits. I always wondered what the thrill of skydiving was. This Mid-Life's Mama's blood pressure may be unable to handle a jump from an airplane, but I'm determined to take some risks- to jump out of my introverted shell and attempt new challenges. Comfortableness is boring. And the beauty of age is that with each passing year, the permission to be one's self increases. I will embrace life and explore as much as this world has to offer.

Day 29

Often we as parents and caregivers tend to lose who "we" are-or who we once were. Today, write down areas in your life that seem dry or stagnant.

Day 30

Write a brief letter to your old self. Start off with, "Dear Former Me..."

Day 31

Write a short letter to yourself in the future- "Dear _______ in the future."

Day 32

What do you admire most about yourself?

Day 33

What is a dream that you have had, that is now lost?

Day 34

What inspires you- gives you motivation or lights your fire? Write about it.

Day 35- Sprinkle today with.......

Renewal and Relaxation

This week focus on your body- take a long bath and soak in the tub, or take an extra-long shower. If you like essential oils, use those too. If you are sore, try a bath in Epsom salt. If it's in your budget, get a massage.

Week 6

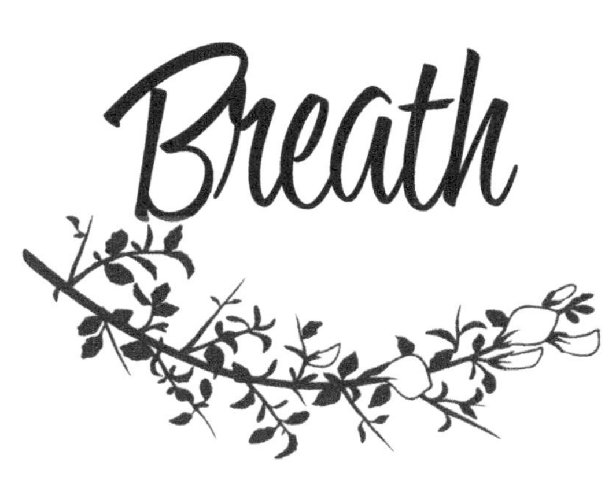

"If oxygen is the only thing you are breathing, then try again. Inhale and soak in everything thing around you and live."

Day 36

As you are reading this, notice your breath. Are you breathing shallow breaths? Is your heart racing? Talk about how you are breathing right now and think about what happened over the past week.

Day 37

What things have an impact on your breathing? Do you find you hold your breath when you are stressed? Write about times when you are stressed & feel smothered.

Day 38

Think about the choices you have had to make in the last month. Have any of them stressed you out? Do you wish you could change anything?

Day 39

Today take 5. Write down 5 things you see with your eyes, 4 things you feel with your hands, 3 things you hear with your ears, 2 things you smell with your nose, and 1 thing you taste with your mouth.

Day 40

Free thoughts- Let your brain wander where it leads you. Write down whatever is on your mind and let your thoughts flow.

Day 41

Think about your happy place. Is it on a beach, or in a cabin in the mountains? Write about the place where you feel most peaceful.

Day 42- Sprinkle today with.......

Yoga

Today work on your breathing by trying Yoga. You don't have to join a class. Simply find videos and engage your body at home.

Week 7

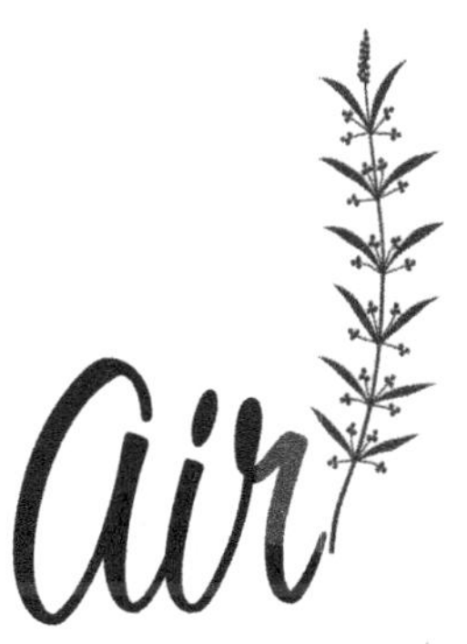

Drowning

Feet first- an airless descent.
With a heavy splash, she enters the water.
The bubbles overtake her head.
They float to the top, as if a means for survival.
She feels the blue water surround her body and soak through her hair.
She asks if this is her destiny.
This sensation of feeling overwhelmed and overtaken by faint whispers of accusations and hidden self-doubt:
"She can do better. She's not a good mom. She'll never get it all done. She needs to discipline her kids. She's doing too much. She needs to clean her house. She needs to lose weight. She doesn't deserve to be a mom..."
These thoughts propel her deeper.
The cause of her sudden plummet off said cliff...
Was it her well-defined, straight-laced definition of motherhood?
Or the social media persecution for her decision to vaccinate.
Or maybe her weekly mom's gathering in which most of the moms proclaimed authoritarianism and complete control over their households and children.
In true Stepford wives fashion, the subtle judgments of other mothers pushed her toward the cliff.
And now she is drowning.
Drowning from the gap between imaginary perfection and life's reality.
She's the mom that works 2 jobs to pay bills, and yet feels guilty for working so much.
She's the mom who holds deep fears that her children will get hurt one day because she is secretly still hurting.
She's the mom who doesn't do well helping her kids on projects and holds questionable cooking skills, but has forgotten how many other things she does do well.
She's the mom of a kid with complex needs, who can't help feeling like it's her fault.
She's the mom whose child just had a complete meltdown, and everyone just stopped and stared.
She's the mom who watches the news and is terrified to send her kids to school because she doesn't know if they will return home safely.

She's drowning in her own guilt and doubt and deeply wishes you would help save her with a little kindness.

Pull her out of the water by voicing a little less judgment (if you see her kid screaming, offer to help and don't just stare).

Pull her up by supporting her well-researched and 6-month-long-final-decision to not vaccinate and homeschool (disagree if you must, but be nice).

Pull her up by saying "Hello" to her child that is nonverbal.

Lift her up by randomly telling her she's a good mom by choosing time with kids, over a museum-like clean house.

Lift her up if she decides she wants a career.

Lift her up if she wants to stay home with her kids.

Organic or non-organic

Breast or bottle

Home school or Private School

Vegetables or Fast Food

Co-sleeping or Cry-it-out

College or Trade School

Gluten-free or Carb-loaded

Lift her up because she is a mother. She loves her kids. She tries equally as hard as you. Her ultimate goal is to have happy, successful kids.

Just.

Like.

You.

If you see her drowning by the weight of the world, by the hard task of parenting, or by the judgments of society-

If you see her bashed on social media or if you see her doubting her mothering skills and abilities...

Promise to save her, lift her up, and refuse to let her drown.

Day 43

Have you felt like you were drowning lately? If so, write about it. Is there anyone in your life who helped you breathe? If so, consider thanking that person.

Day 44

Today write about the air around you, or the atmosphere. Is your home life pleasant and calm, or rocky and stressful?

Day 45

Today, if you work outside of your home, write about the air there. Is your work environment stressful too? Are there people at work who change the atmosphere of your job? Is there anything you could do differently to change the air?

Day 46

Mentally, how is your air? Do you have an air of stress, resentment, negativity, or pessimism? Or do you feel like you exude the feelings of positivity, patience, and optimism?

Day 47

As you reread my article about drowning, think about the negative statements you have heard about being a mom or caretaker. What kind of negative statements run through your head?

Day 48

What are your deepest fears about the person you take care of? Do those fears impact your behavior?

Day 49- Sprinkle today with.......

Air

Today focus on the air around you. Look for videos on Guided Mediation or Guided Imagery. Focus on changing your atmosphere and being present and in the moment.

Week 8

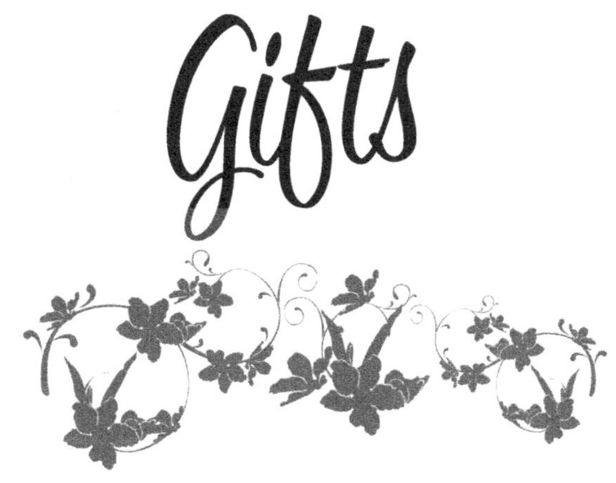

"You are gifted far beyond what you know-
embrace and allow your talents to grow."

Day 50

Today write down every area in which you are gifted. Don't be shy. You are beautiful and full of so much potential.

Day 51

In what ways do you share your gifts and talents? Do you share them on a daily basis?

Day 52

Most people have more than one talent. What gifts do you have others do not know about? Is there anything that hinders you from sharing your gifts?

Day 53

If you could do anything with your gifts and talents, what would you do?

Day 54

Are there any gifts and talents you wish you didn't have? Or is there a part of your gifts that sometimes feel like a burden or hardship? Write about it.

Day 55

Think about your talent or gifts. What is a way your gift could impact the world? Would it be possible to share your gift in that way?

Day 56- Sprinkle today with.......

Your Gift

Today's a daring day. Take a chance and share your talent with someone else- maybe a trusted individual. If you are feeling extra bold, do a live video on social media and talk about or share your talent!

Week 9

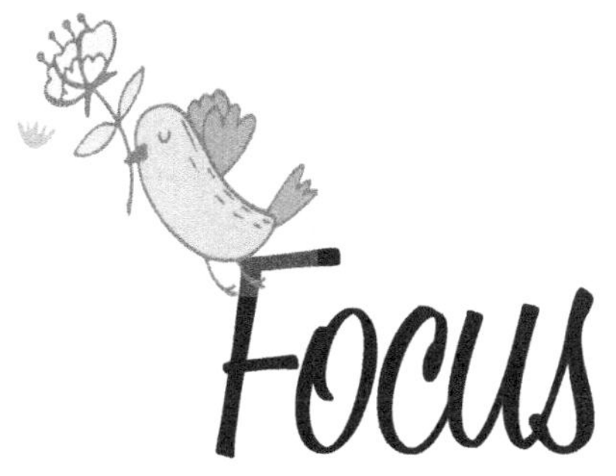

Focus

"Focus is being patient and not talking so much."

-Ella, 5 yrs. old

Day 57

This week the focus is on you. Write down your deepest fears.

Day 58

What is your biggest worry right now you can't seem to get rid of?

Day 59

Let's try some light-hearted thoughts. The rest of the week is for fun. Today- write down a list of books that are amazing, and then list books that are garbage.

Day 60

Write down your list of must-see movies/tv series. Be sure to share it with your friends or Facebook group. See if they agree.

Day 61

Think about your home and what's in it. If you could, what changes would you make? The color? Would you move? Plant flowers?

Day 62

Write down a list of meals that you absolutely love. List your favorite recipes too. Make a list of dishes you want to try in the future.

Day 63- Sprinkle today with.......

Focus

Today- spend a few hours on YOU! Watch a movie in quiet- take a nap- get a pedicure. Today you must spend time (even if it is only a few hours) focusing on YOU and what YOU would like to do.

Week 10

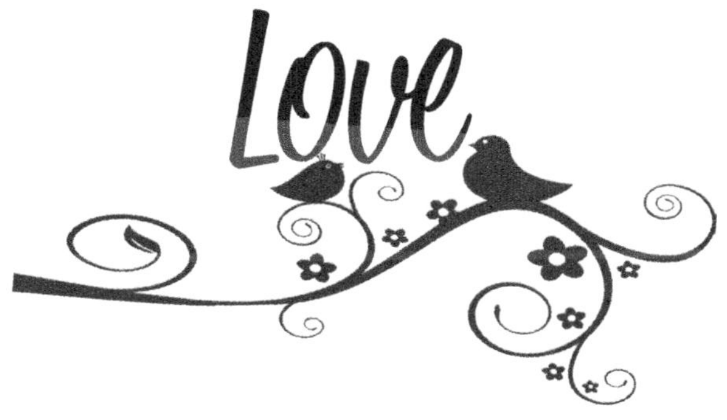

Letter to Ella

I breathed a bit easier on the day you were born.
From my over-stretched, worn-out belly you emerged, with a mezzo-soprano scream.
You were my rainbow baby, almost 2 years after my miscarriage.
When I heard the Doctor say, "She's fine," I felt at ease.

It wasn't that I feared Down Syndrome, it was that I felt concerned about all the medical complications that sometimes go along with Down Syndrome. Your older sister was born with Down Syndrome, and it was a shock to me because I had no idea about her extra chromosome until she was born.

I've loved your sister since her birth, just as I love you, but I've hated seeing her deal with medical problems... the surgeries... sleepless nights.
And so daddy and I prayed for a healthy baby.
And so you were.

As I write this letter to my sweet neurotypical daughter Ella,
I hope you realize you were never meant for a life of normalcy because you were not born under normal circumstances, or in a normal atmosphere.
Your older sister with Down Syndrome has helped create our beautiful, fabulously unique, "abnormal" atmosphere. She has filled our home with immeasurable love and joy, and you have made our joy complete.

Ella,
Your older sister Tayler has a unique gift, although others may not view it as such. She has a gift of love, which often causes her to go against the grain and share it with the world. I do believe my sweet girl, that you have this gift as well. I've watched as you have run up to "Sissy" and hang tightly to her leg. With your simple "I love you Tayler Beth," you have caused the room to permeate with love. I've never said the words "Down Syndrome" to you and I doubt you know what they mean. All you appear to know is that Sissy is awesome.
Mommy agrees.

Tayler has had a lot of difficulty talking over the years and using sign language has never really been an option for us because of her fine motor skills. So I often wondered how you girls would communicate once you began to talk. I'm amazed Ella, at the way you interact with your sister. You speak to her without expectation of return.

I love when you voluntarily give her a kiss or have giggle time with her. You've always shown so much respect for her and you have never left your sister Tayler behind. I've observed when you get your sister's clothes or glasses to help her prepare for school. Mom loves how you are especially concerned when she is feeling ill and has to go to the doctor. Full of empathy you are, Mommy could not have dreamed of a more beautiful baby sister.

Ella, As you grow into a teen, I hope you understand that you will rarely be treated equally. Please know that mommy and daddy are not being unfair or mean we just have different requirements for you both. And though our love for you will always be equal, our requirements will not be.

Because you are a fast learner Ella, Daddy and I will challenge you. We will challenge you, not to hurt you, but similar to sister's language barrier, we will challenge you to break barriers. We will push your older sister Tayler to do the same, however, this push may look slightly different. Just know that it's for your good.

And as you get older, mommy and daddy do have an expectation that you will be patient not only with your sister, but with others like her, or others with disabilities. And on days where your patience fails, we will show you a video of your 2-year-old tantrum. We will remind you that to whom much is given, much is required.

I want to warn you that you will learn as you grow that there are horribly mean people in the world. They may make fun of your sister. They will stare. I hope you can be brave enough to defend her if mommy and daddy are not around. And if you find yourself feeling embarrassed or at a loss for words, mommy won't be angry. We will talk about it and develop a plan to address it for next time. All we ask is that you continue to show your sister love, just as we and your sister have always shown you.

Day 64

You have spent the last several weeks focused on your feelings about your role as a caregiver. This week, focus on your other family members. Write down the names of each person in your family and share 2 qualities you love about that person.

Day 65

Today share about the best times you have had as a family together.

Day 66

As caregivers, we often unintentionally neglect our on needs. Write how you ensure you spend special time with other members of your family. Share how you will spend purposeful time with other family members in the future.

Are there any ways you wish your family could show more love to each other?

Day 68

What are your hopes and wishes for other members of your family?

Day 69

If your family includes other children, how have you planned for them? Do you have strategic financial plans?

Day 70- Sprinkle today with.......

Love

Today- schedule fun time with each other person in your family. And if you are a sole caretaker, schedule time with a friend. Be sure to let that person know what you love about them and what makes them special!

Week 11

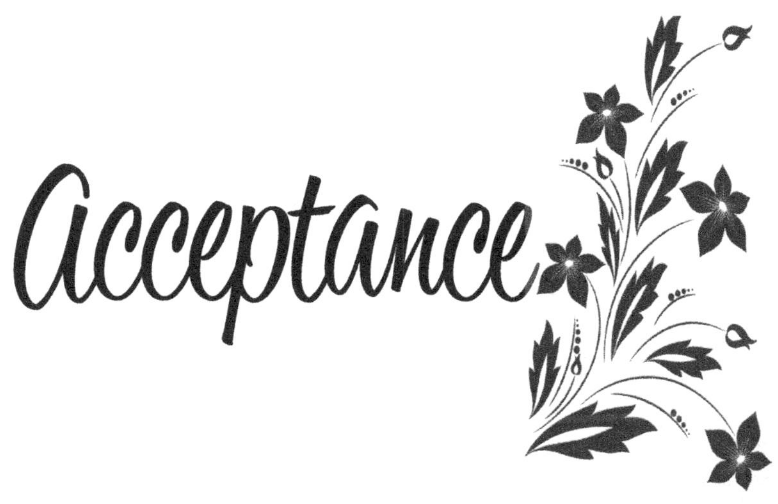

Finding Peace

11 years to be exact. I hope you don't judge me, but it really did take me awhile.
The road to serenity... full of dips, turns, and sometimes treacherous curves.
I have thoughts as to why it took so long for me. Maybe it was because my daughter was non-verbal. I kept waiting for her words to spew out and flood my life. But it has yet to happen.
Receiving a diagnosis of Down Syndrome, or any unexpected diagnosis can be metamorphic. It's as if one's brain must race to catch up to an impending, befuddled uncertainty.
Medical professionals are required to give patients knowledge, or the "reality" if you will. It's up to the patient to determine what he or she will do with this knowledge.
It took 11 years before I was able to merge "reality" with my "hopes and prayers" to deliver my current level of peace.
Here are the nonlinear, 6 Steps I took to reach peace with my daughter's diagnosis.

1. I Cried.

A whole lot. In the many hospitals. At the doctor's office. After birthday parties. After IEP meetings. I hurt not because of lack of love, but because she was different. I was well aware of how the world treats those who are different.
I thought the tears were defeatist and showed my weakness as a mom. I didn't know their healing power. Those tears were a release. A salve to my wounded heart.

2. I Read.

A lot. Anything that I could find related to sign language, hypothyroidism, and Down Syndrome. I read any book on Sensory Integration that I could find. I researched therapies. I even did the dreaded medical Google searches, searching for a cause.... Even a cure. The more I read, the more I learned that no one could really define my daughter because every child with Down Syndrome is different.

3. I acknowledged my fear.

Deep down, I was very afraid. How could my non-verbal child (now a teen) survive in a world that thrives on verbal communication? Was she angry because she lacked the ability to express herself? How would she ever work? Would she ever be truly independent? So...Back to number 1.
More tears from the conversations we may never have.
I acknowledged my fear with the clause to do something about it. I then...

4. Started Writing

Tucked on a dusty bookshelf are the beginnings of my memoir. I'm an Introvert. My home is my sanctuary. I'm not naturally "peoplely." Joining a Down Syndrome support group was somewhat counterintuitive for me because of my personality. So I started writing. Writing was my release and my therapy. I was able to express and share my story so that other parents could have confirmation.

5. I found love.

As cliché as it sounds, it was my happy beginning. I met my husband 7 years ago. He represented the epitome of calm and peace, from my somewhat chaotic, un-predictable life. He promised to love my sweet daughter as his own.

And he still does.

And when 1 & 2 occur I have his support and advice. Or if there is no advice, I at least have a hug.

6. I let go of guilt.

It's not my fault. 11 years and I know. I wanted and prayed for a healthy baby throughout my pregnancy. I received a healthy baby, even though it took us longer to reach health. She may not be complete or perfect by the world's definition, but she is wonderfully made to me.

So, how can you find peace with a medical diagnosis? Here are my suggestions:

- Cry when you must.

Feel what you feel. Let your tears fuel your fire to advocate and fight for your child.

- Fight fear with research and exploration.

Ask questions. Don't accept every answer. Use your intuition. Get a second and third opinion. Then make a plan. And if that plan doesn't work, create a new one.

- Discover what motivates you and gives you release.

Take time for you. Find a hobby or something you enjoy doing. Take care of yourself. Laugh. A lot. Even when it hurts.

- Use support

Find someone who loves your child just as much as you do. It doesn't have to be a spouse. It can be a friend or trusted neighbor. Even if they can't "fix" it, at least open up and talk to someone. And if words don't come, just try a hug. It really is powerful.

Even if finding peace takes you 11 years, it can happen.

Day 71

When is the last time you cried? Write about it. Does it still make you sad?

Day 72

What is the latest research on your loved one's medical conditions? Are you optimistic about it? Do you have access to this innovation?

Day 73

What secret fears do you have you have not yet acknowledged?

Day 74

I know you already like to write, but what other outlets do you have to share your feelings? Are you in any social media or community support groups? If you are not, would you be willing to join? Write down a few groups you could participate in.

Day 75

Do you have anyone in your circle or on your social media pages who just have too much negativity? Who is it and how can you avoid that negativity?

Day 76

What might your future look like with your loved one? What does your own future look like? Have you accepted what your future may look like? Write more about it.

Day 77- Sprinkle today with.......

Acceptance

Today spend time with someone who is now in your support group (physically or on the Internet). Maybe a phone call, a video chat, or better yet- in person!

Week 12

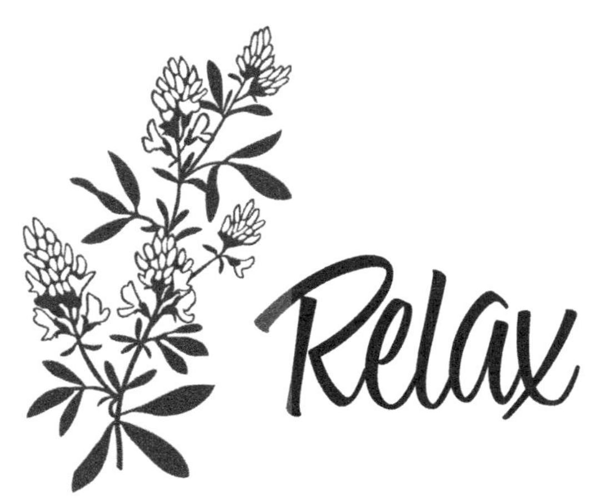

"If chill really were available in a pill-
I'd want a patch!"

Day 78

Every day this week will bring an actionable step. 1st up-get out and walk! Research shows exercise is a powerful weapon against physical disease and depression. Enough talk- get out and walk! When finished, write about your experience!

Day 79

Today is easy. Download a relaxation app. There are tons of apps to help you relax. Once you have chosen one, get busy and complete at least one activity. When you finish, share how the activity made you feel.

Day 80

Find a video on progressive muscle relaxation. Do it. Don't just put this journal down. Go do it. And then write about it.

Day 81

Today- get the whole family (or a friend). BOTH of you complete an exercise together on guided imagery. Make everyone feel relaxed and calm.

Day 82

Today find a few videos on deep breathing, as you did a few weeks ago. Be sure to focus and remain present.

Day 83

Today stretch your body. If you are unsure of what to do... well you already know now- find a video.

Day 84- Sprinkle today with.......

More Relaxation

Today is easy. Reflect back on your week. Write down how you can find at least ONE way you can relax each week. Then schedule it. On your phone or in your planner.

Week 13

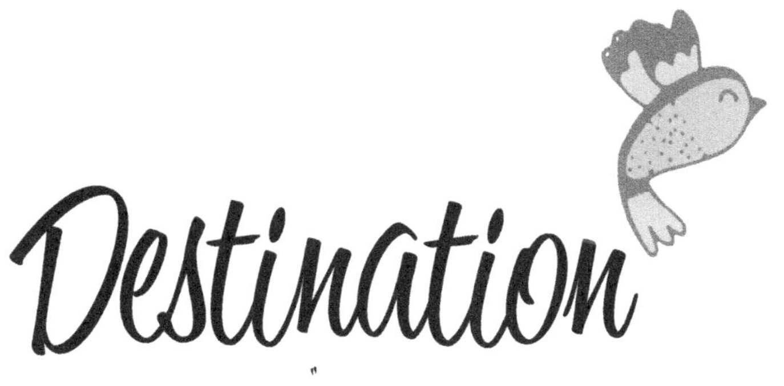

"Accept that your life won't look like everyone else's. But that won't mean it's not beautiful."

You have spent the last few weeks purposefully spending time on you. I am proud of you. During this final week- let's focus on your future. Some of it will be hard, but I promise you it is very necessary.

Day 85

Will you be a forever caregiver like me? Have you thought about what you would do if something happened to you?

Day 86

Have you made plans financially for the future? What other steps do you need to take? Are you even able to think about it at this moment?

Day 87

What possible additional supports will your loved one need in the future?

Day 88

What are your thoughts now about your loved one's future? Be honest with yourself and share them.

Day 89

Do you compare your life with others? Have you ever been jealous of other's life? What ideas and comparisons do you need to throw away?

Day 90

Write about how you can embrace and take one day at a time.

Day 91- Sprinkle today with.......

Your Destination

On day one, we shared how your caregiver journey began. Now let's talk about how your caregiver journey will continue and what the future will hold. Talk about past victories and how you plan to celebrate future victories.

By now, I hope you feel a bit refreshed. I hope your blades are finally beginning to flourish and that you are hopeful and full of a little joy. Remember to water your grass- and that it is okay to spend time for you. Recognize the lows and hard parts, but be sure to enjoy life's beautiful moments. You have permission to slow down.

Take the time to truly live.

Favorite Relaxation Videos

Favorite Relaxation Apps

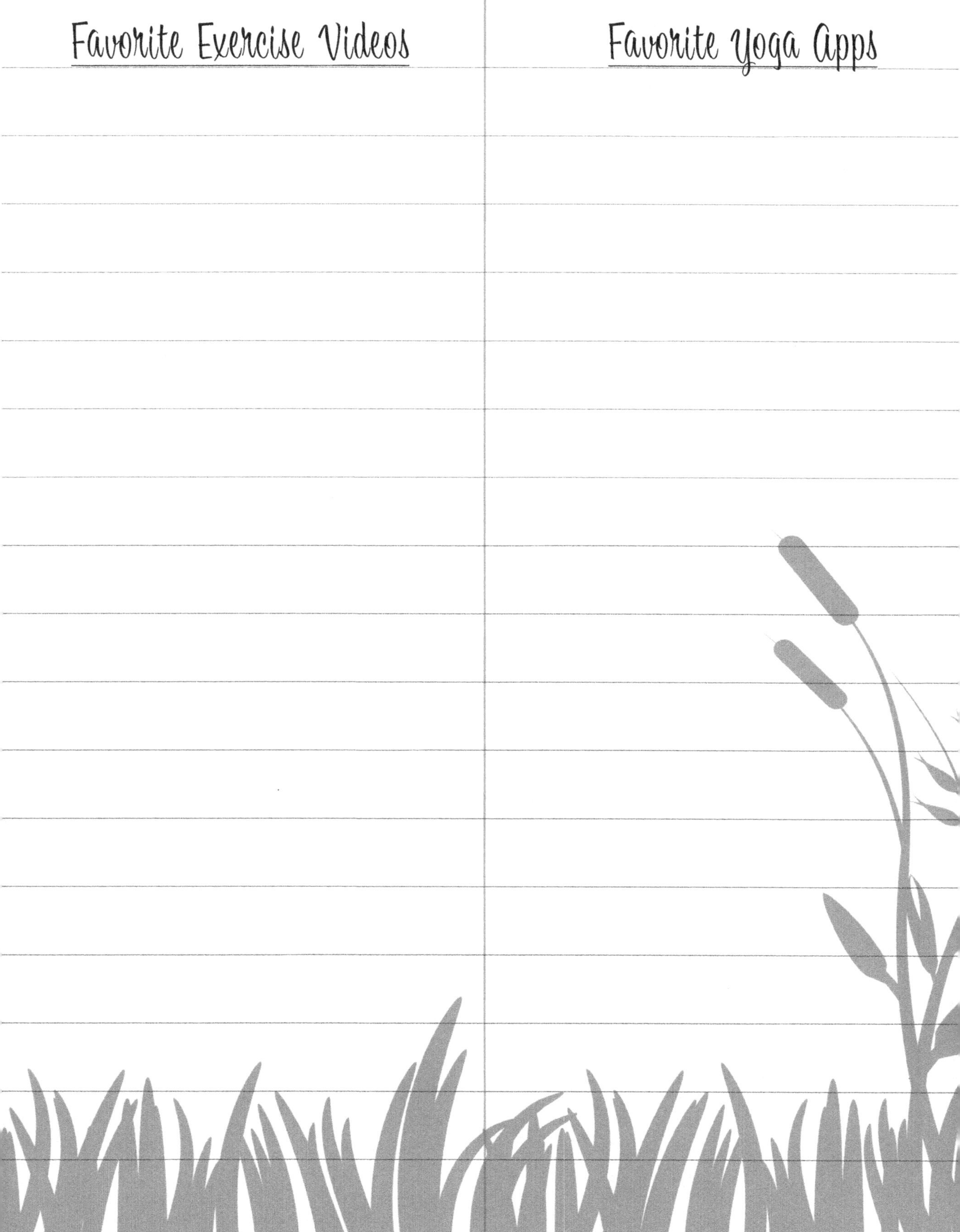
Favorite Exercise Videos
Favorite Yoga Apps

To Do:

To Do:

Important!

Important!

Notes

Notes

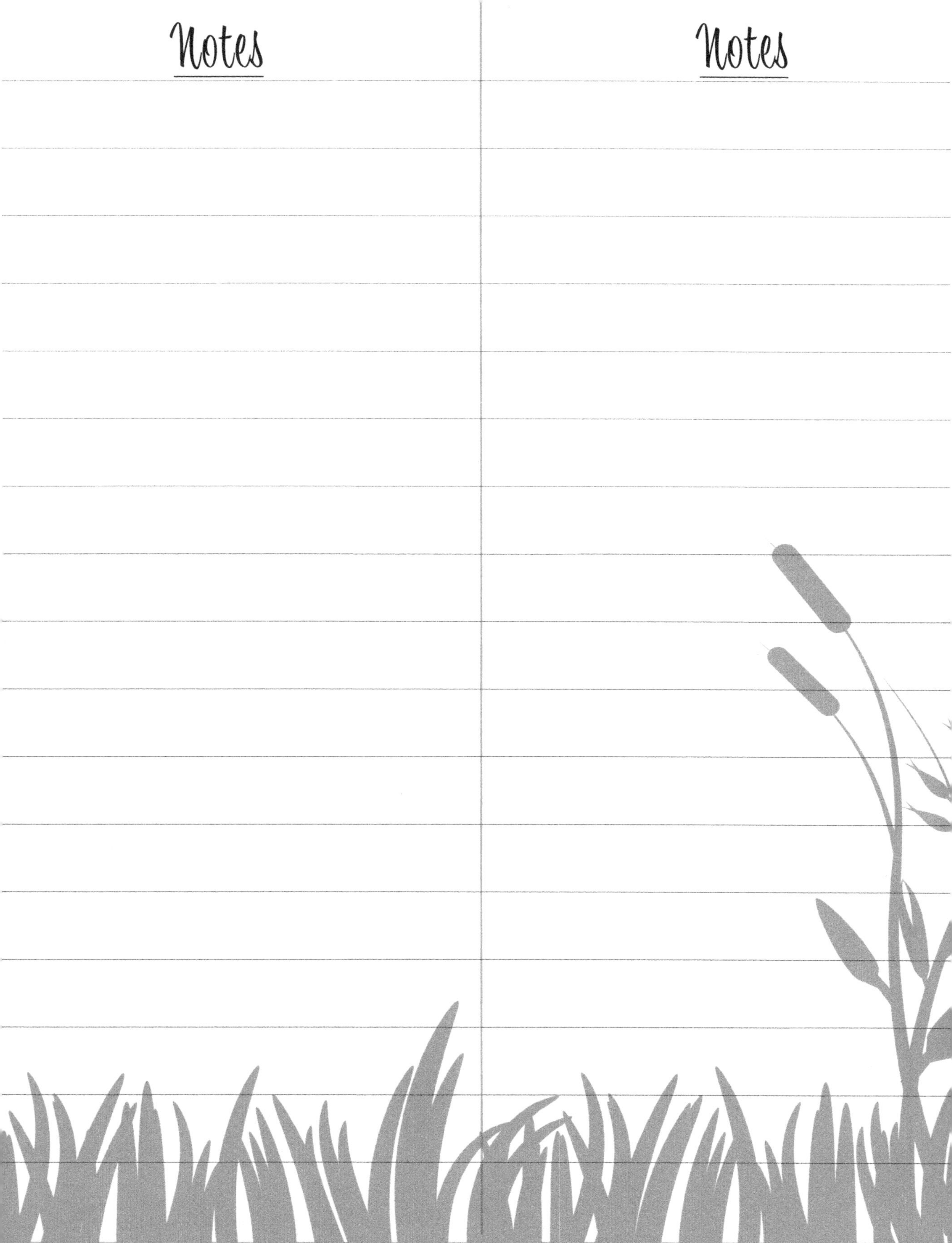
Notes
Notes

Made in the USA
Monee, IL
20 August 2020

38811505R00072